# LOW-SODIUM
# COOKBOOK

*Flavorful and simple low-sodium recipes for a healthier*

*meal-plan*

## MC Cooking Academy

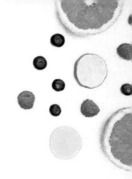

# Table of Content

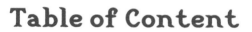
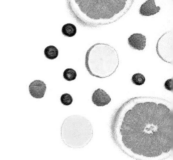

# BREAKFAST RECIPES

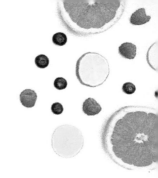

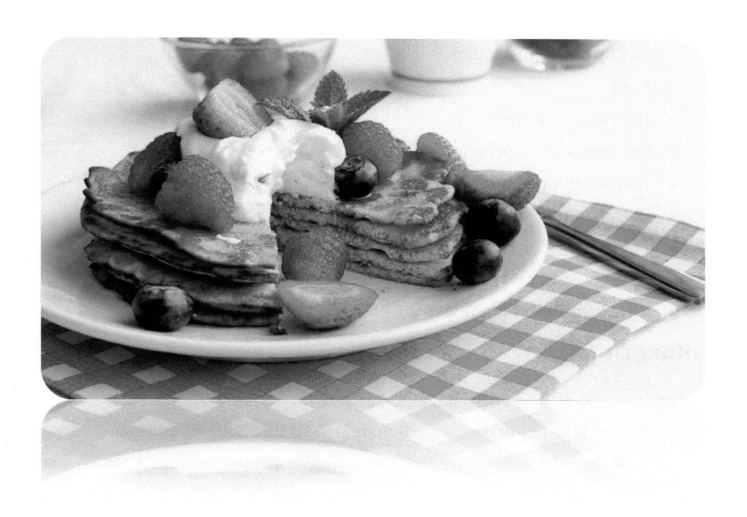

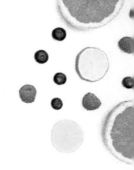

# Feta Cheese and eggs Breakfast

Prep Time: 5 Minutes | Cooking Time: 10 Minutes | Servings: 3

## INGREDIENTS:

- ¼ Cup of chopped sweet red pepper
- ¼ Cup of chopped onion
- 1 egg
- 1/8 Teaspoon of salt
- 1/8 Teaspoon of pepper
- 1 Small chopped tomato
- ½ Cup of torn fresh baby spinach
- 1 to ½ teaspoons of minced fresh basil
- 2 Pita breads
- 2 Tablespoons of crumbled feta cheese

## DIRECTIONS:

1. In a medium non-stick skillet greased with cooking spray, cook the red pepper and the onion over a medium high heat for about 3 minutes
2. Add in the egg substitute, the salt and the pepper and cook until your ingredients are set
3. Mix the spinach, the tomato and the basil; then spoon it over the pitas; then top with the egg mixture
4. Sprinkle with the feta cheese
5. Serve and enjoy your breakfast!

# NUTRITION

Kcal: 267

Fat: 4

Carbs: 6

Proteins: 3

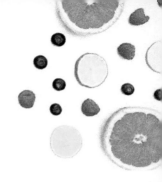

# Hummus With veggies breakfast

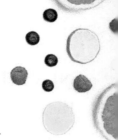

Prep Time: 10 Minutes | Cooking Time: 10 Minutes | Servings: 3-4

**INGREDIENTS:**

- 1 Tablespoon of avocado oil or of olive oil
- 1 Pound of asparagus, chopped into pieces and with the ends trimmed
- 3 Cups of shredded kale leaves
- 1 Batch of lemony dressing
- 3 Cups of shredded (uncooked) Brussels sprouts
- 1 and ½ cups of cooked quinoa
- ½ Cup of hummus
- 1 Peeled, pitted and thinly-sliced avocado
- 4 Large cooked eggs
- For the garnishes: Sliced almonds; sunflower seeds and crushed red pepper

For the Lemon dressing:

- 2 Tablespoons of avocado oil or of olive oil
- 2 Tablespoons of freshly-squeezed lemon juice
- 2 Teaspoons of Dijon mustard
- 1 Minced garlic clove
- 1 Pinch of salt and freshly-cracked black pepper

**DIRECTIONS:**

TO MAKE THE BREAKFAST BOWLS:

1. Start by heating the oil in a large sauté pan over a medium-high heat; then add in the asparagus and sauté for about 4 to 5 minutes and stir from time to time

2. Remove from the heat; then set aside

3. Combine the lemony dressing with the kale and massage the dressing with your fingers into the kale for about 2 to 3 minutes

4. Add in the Brussels sprouts, the quinoa, and the cooked asparagus; then toss until your ingredients are very well combined.

5. To assemble your ingredients, divide the kale salad evenly between the bowls; then top with the avocado, the egg and your favorite garnishes

TO MAKE THE LEMON VINAIGRETTE:

6. Whisk all your ingredients together in a large mixing bowl until your ingredients are very well combined.

7. Serve and enjoy your breakfast!

**NUTRITION**

Kcal: 89.5

Fat: 2.8

Carbs: 14.1

Proteins: 4.3

# Breakfast Burritos

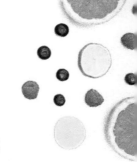

Prep Time: 10 Minutes | Cooking Time: 5 Minutes | Servings: 6

## INGREDIENTS

- 6 Whole tortillas, sun dried
- 9 Whole eggs
- 2 Cups of washed and dried baby spinach
- 3 Tablespoons of sliced black olives
- 3 Tablespoons of chopped sun-dried tomatoes
- ½ Cup of feta cheese
- ¾ Cup of canned refried beans

## DIRECTIONS:

1. Start by spraying a medium frying pan with a non- stick cooking spray.
2. Scramble the eggs and toss it for about 5 minutes, or until the eggs become no longer liquid
3. Add the spinach, the black olives, the sun-dried tomatoes and stir
4. Add in the Feta cheese and cover until the cheese is completely melted
5. Add in 2 tablespoons of refried beans to each of the tortillas.
6. Top with the egg mixture and divide evenly between all the burritos.
7. Wrap your tortillas; then rill on a Panini press or in a frying pan
8. Serve and enjoy with a salsa of your choice!

## NUTRITION

Kcal: 252

Fat: 11

Carbs: 21

Proteins: 14

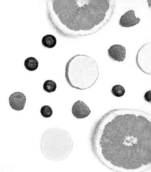

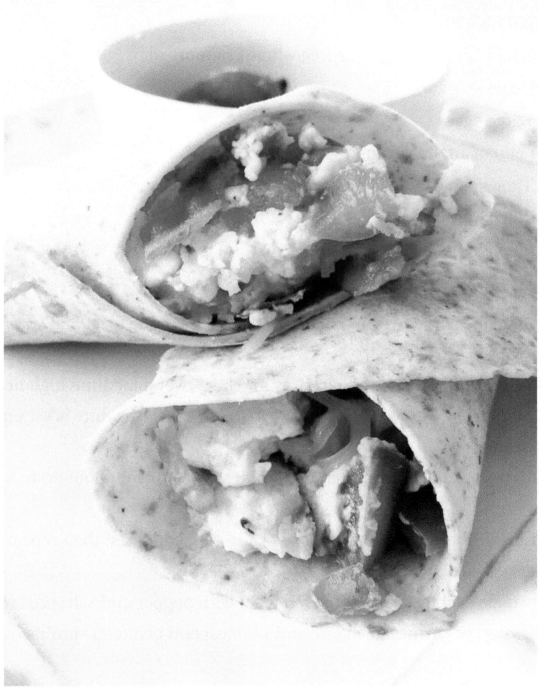

# Avocado Toast

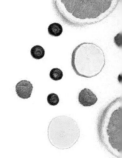

Prep Time: 10 Minutes | Cooking Time: 5 Minutes | Servings: 6

## INGREDIENTS:

- 4 Slices of toasted, gluten-free whole grain bread
- 1 Large avocado
- 4 Large eggs
- ¼ cup of alfalfa sprouts
- 2 Tablespoons of freshly shaved parmesan cheese
- 1 Pinch of salt
- 1 Pinch of pepper

## DIRECTIONS:

1. Divide the sliced avocado between the pieces of the toast and spread on top of the bread
2. Spray a skillet with cooking spray and heat over a medium high heat
3. Crack an egg into your skillet and cook until the egg white is set on the bottom
4. Flip the egg to cook on each of the sides perfectly for about 30 to 45 seconds
5. Transfer the cooked egg to the avocado-topped toasts; then repeat until all the eggs are cooked
6. Sprinkle each of the egg covered toast with pepper and salt; the layer shavings of parmesan cheese and 1 tablespoon of alfalfa sprouts over the top
7. Serve and enjoy your Breakfast!

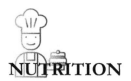

# NUTRITION

Kcal: 189

Fat: 11

Carbs: 20

Proteins: 3.6

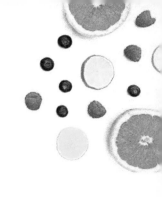

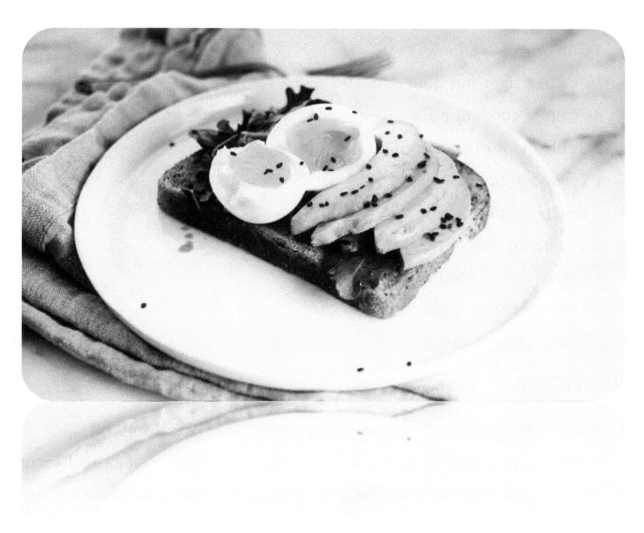

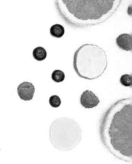

# Banana coconut Pancakes

Prep Time: 10 Minutes | Cooking Time: 10 Minutes | Servings: 4

## INGREDIENTS

- 2 Medium ripe bananas
- 1 Cup of cassava flour
- ½ Cup of tiger nut flour
- ¾ Cup of coconut milk
- 2 Tablespoons of coconut oil
- 1 Teaspoon of baking soda
- 1 Teaspoon of sea salt
- 2 Teaspoon of ground cinnamon
- 1 Cup of fresh blueberries
- 1 Tablespoon of apple cider vinegar
- 2 Tablespoons of coconut oil

## DIRECTIONS:

1. Mix all of your ingredients very well, except for the coconut oil
2. Place 1 teaspoon of oil into a large nonstick saucepan over a medium heat.
3. When the oil starts melting; spoon about tablespoons of the batter; then shape it with a spoon into pancakes of round shape
4. Cook the pancake for about 3 to 5 minutes per side; then flip the pancakes when the edges get a brown color.
5. Serve and enjoy your pancakes!

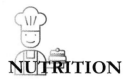

# NUTRITION

Kcal: 149.4

Fat: 13.2

Carbs: 4.52

Proteins: 6.3

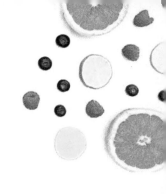

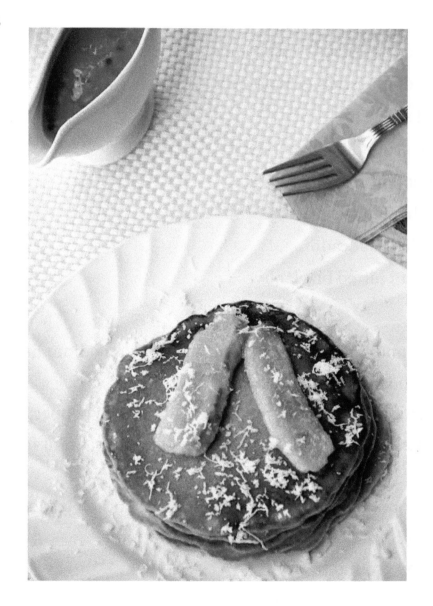

# Ground meat Hash browns with mushrooms

Prep Time: 6 Minutes | Cooking Time: 10 Minutes | Servings: 3-4

## INGREDIENTS

- 1 Medium, sliced onion
- 6 To 8 medium, sliced mushrooms
- ½ Pound of grass-fed ground beef
- 1 Pinch of salt
- 1 Pinch of ground black pepper
- ½ Teaspoon of smoked paprika
- 2 Lightly beaten eggs
- 1 Small, diced avocado
- 10 sliced and pitted black olives

## DIRECTIONS:

1. In a heavy and large non-stick wok and over a medium heat, melt a small 1 or 2 tablespoons of coconut oil
2. Add the onions, the mushrooms, the salt and the pepper; then cook the ingredients until your veggies become soft and fragrant for about 3 minutes
3. Add the ground beef and the smoked paprika; then let cook for about 7 minutes or until the beef meat is no longer pink
4. Remove the ground beef
5. Add the eggs to the wok and mix to scramble it
6. Return the beef to your wok and add the sliced olives and the avocado
7. Cook your ingredients for about 40 seconds
8. Transfer your breakfast to a serving dish

9. Garnish your breakfast with parsley; then serve and enjoy!

10. Transfer to a pretty bowl, garnish with parsley if desired, sit yourself down and enjoy

**NUTRITION**

Kcal: 230

Fat: 15

Carbs: 6

Proteins: 22

# Scotch Eggs breakfast

Prep Time: 10 Minutes | Cooking Time: 10 Minutes | Servings: 6-7

## INGREDIENTS:

- 6 to 7 medium eggs
- 1 Pound of ground beef
- 1 Tablespoon of homemade gingerbread spice
- 1 and ½ teaspoons of salt
- ½ Teaspoon of black pepper
- 1 Tablespoon of honey

## DIRECTIONS:

1. Hard boil the eggs into 2 cups of water in a saucepan for about 7 to 10 minutes or you can also steam it because it makes removing the shells of the eggs easier.

2. Preheat your oven to a temperature of about 350°F; then Line a baking sheet with a parchment paper.

3. Take a deep and large bowl; then combine the ground meat, the ginger spice, the salt, the pepper and the honey

4. Arrange the eggs over a tray; then fill about 1/3 cup of the meat mixture and make it lump with your hands

5. Flatten the beef meat and place an egg into the center

6. Fold the meat around the egg and gently flatten it until you cover the entire egg

7. Repeat the same process with the remaining eggs and once you finish; arrange the eggs over your already prepared baking sheet

8. Bake your scotch eggs in the oven for about 20 minutes

9. Remove the eggs from the oven and set it aside to cool for about 5 minutes

10. Serve and enjoy your scotch eggs!

**NUTRITION**

Kcal: 168.6

Fat: 8.1

Carbs: 2

Proteins: 23

# FISH AND SEAFOOD RECIPES

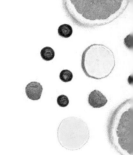

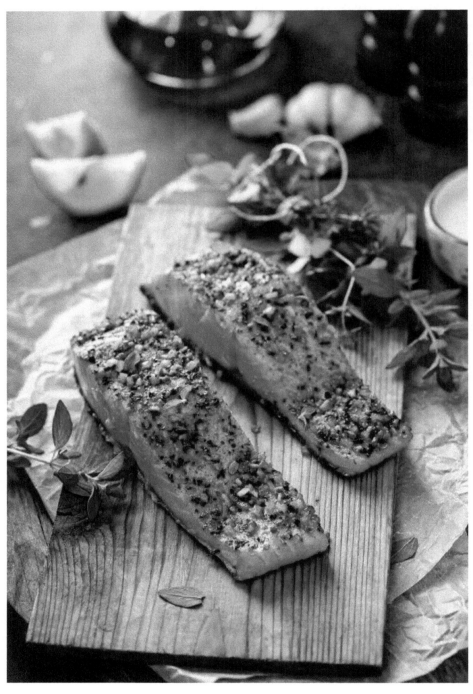

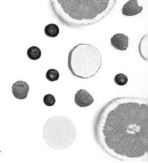

# Halibut fish with lemon and paprika

Prep Time: 8 minutes| Cooking Time: 10 Minutes| Servings: 4

## INGREDIENTS

- 4 Cups of packed spinach
- 2 Halibut fish meat of 11oz each
- The Juice of half a lemon
- 1 Pinch of salt
- 1 Pinch of pepper
- 1 Pinch of smoked paprika
- 1 sliced lemon
- Sliced green onions
- 1 Deseeded and thinly sliced red chili
- 1 Cup of halved cherry tomatoes
- 2 tbsp of avocado oil

## DIRECTIONS

1. Place two squares of the same size of halibut fish over a flat surface
2. Divide the spinach between the squares
3. Place the halibut over a chopping board; then remove the membrane and the bone
4. You should have about 5 pieces all in all
5. Lay the first 2 pieces of halibut over each of the spinach piles; then squeeze the lemon over each part

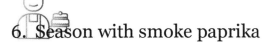

6. Season with smoke paprika

7. Top with lemon slices

8. Top each fillet with the sliced green onions, the chili and the cherry tomatoes

9. Pour 1 tbsp of avocado oil over each fish portion

10. Tightly wrap the foil around the fish; then arrange the two in the flat pan

11. Leave to cook for 10 minutes

12. Remove when the fish turns into gold

13. Serve and enjoy your dish!

14. You can use sesame oil instead of avocado oil and use salmon instead of halibut.

**NUTRITION**

Kcal: 299

Fat: 9.5

Carbs: 8.3

 Proteins: 2

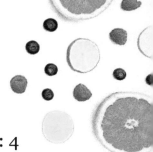

# Fish-stuffed Cucumber

Prep Time: 10 minutes| Cooking Time: 10 Minutes| Servings: 4

## INGREDIENTS

- 4 cucumbers
- ½ pound of cod or other white fish
- 2 organic eggs
- 1 lemon
- 1 Greek yogurt
- 1 Pinch salt and pepper

## DIRECTIONS:

1. Blanch the cucumbers in salted boiling water for 10 minutes.
2. Cut in half to dig them.
3. Cut the fish into pieces, mix with the eggs and yogurt, season; add the chopped cucumber flesh.
4. Stuff the cucumbers with this mixture and cook in the oven for 10 minutes on slices of lemon.
5. Once the time is up; turn the oven and set aside to cool
6. Serve and enjoy!

## NUTRITION

Kcal: 268.6

Fat: 21.7

Carbs: 11.4

Proteins: 13.2

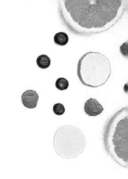
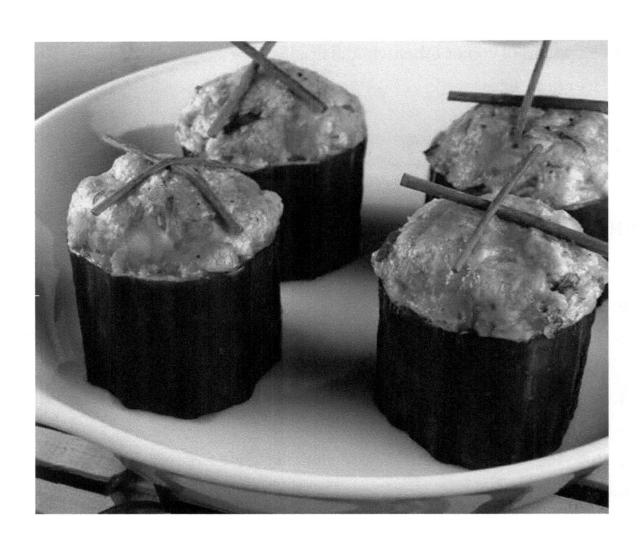

# Smoked Trout Recipe

Prep Time: 10 minutes| Cooking Time: 3 Hours| Servings: 3

## INGREDIENTS:

- 4 To 5 pounds of trout fillets or lake trout fillets, about 8 filets
- 2 Quarts of filtered water
- ½ Cup of kosher salt
- ½ Cup of brown sugar

## DIRECTIONS:

1. Start by removing the pin bones from the trout fillets.
2. Combine the sugar with the salt all together with the water in a large container, about 1 to 2 gallon size; then stir very well until the salt
3. Submerge the trout fillets into the brine and cover the container; then refrigerate for about 3 to 8 hours
4. Remove the trout from the brine; then rinse under running water and remove any excess of moisture from the fillet with clean paper towels; then place the trout fillet with the skin side down over a cooling rack that is fitted in a sheet pan
5. Put the pan in the refrigerator for about 2 hours; up to an overnight
6. Remove 2 racks from your Grill; then place the fillets over the racks with the skin side down; then let the fish rest while you are preparing your Grill
7. Fill the water bowl half way; then place the wood chips into the tray
8. Use alder, oak or maple woodchips; then open the top vent and turn the smoker; preheat to about 160°F

9. Place the racks with the fish in a smoker; then smoke the trout for about 3 hours; replenish the wood chips and the water every about 60 minutes

10. Serve the smoked fish with the toasted baguette slices and with a refreshing green salad

**NUTRITION**

Kcal: 90

Fat: 4.5

Carbs: 2

Proteins: 12

# APPETIZER RECIPES

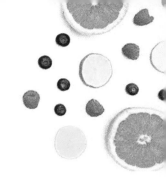

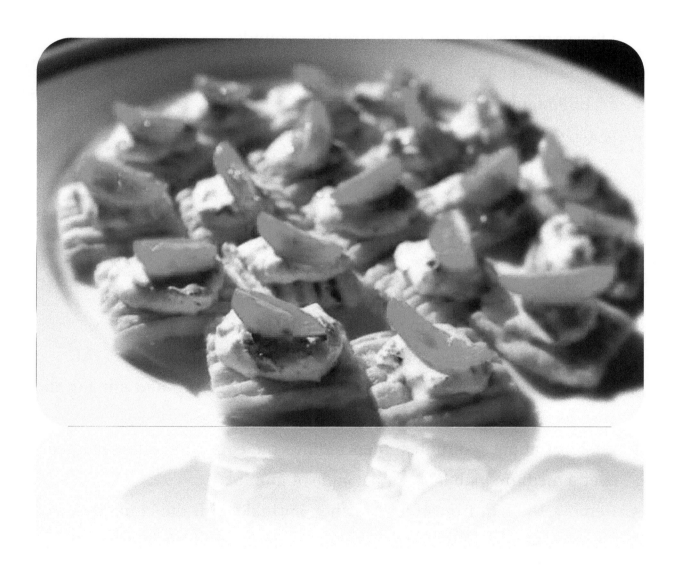

# Glazed Roasted Carrots

Prep Time: 5 minutes| Cooking Time: 8 Minutes| Servings: 3-4

## INGREDIENTS:

- 1 lb carrots, peeled and diced into thick rounds
- 2 TBSP oil, melted
- 2 TBSP maple syrup
- ½ tsp Orange, zest
- ¼ Cup orange, juiced
- ¼ tsp salt
- 1 Pinch cinnamon

## DIRECTIONS:

1. Start by melting the oil in a medium pan
2. Add in the carrots and sauté for about 3 to 4 minutes
3. Pour in the orange juice and add in the maple syrup and stir for about 1 additional minute then cover the pan
4. Cook for about 3 minutes; then remove the cover and simmer uncovered over a medium high heat for a couple of minutes
5. Remove the pan from the heat; then sprinkle with the cinnamon and the orange zest
6. Serve and enjoy your glazed carrots!

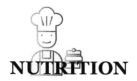

# NUTRITION

Kcal: 157

Fat: 7.6

Carbs: 10

Proteins: 3.1

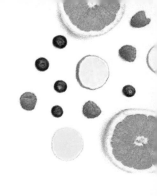

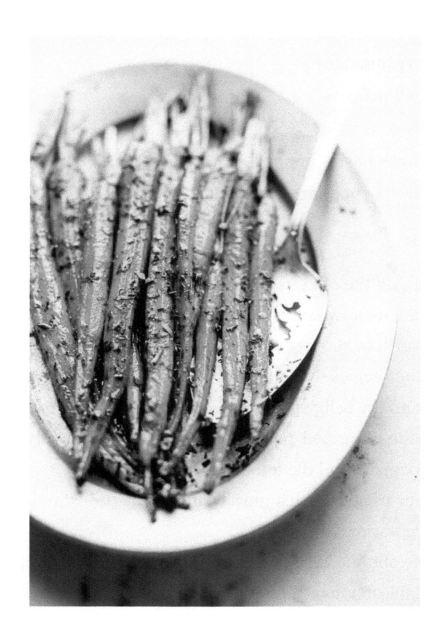

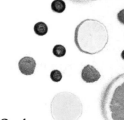

# Roasted Okra

Prep Time: 5 minutes| Cooking Time: 8 Minutes| Servings: 3-4

## INGREDIENTS:

- 1 lb fresh okra, trimmed
- ¼ lb cherry tomatoes
- 3 Green bell peppers
- 2 TBSP olive oil
- ½ TBSP fresh basil, chopped
- 1 Pinch black pepper, freshly ground

## DIRECTIONS:

1. After cleaning the okra, wash the tomatoes and peppers; then combine all the ingredients together in a large mixing bowl
2. Preheat a grill to about 350° F
3. Arrange the veggies over the grill and grill it for about 3 minutes; then turn the okra and the bell peppers and grill for about 2 to 3 additional minutes
4. Transfer the okra, bell peppers and tomatoes to a serving dish and peel both the peppers and the tomatoes
5. Pound your veggies with a mortar and pestle or just pulse the mixture to a food processor or a blender
6. Season the obtained veggie mixture with salt and pepper; then drizzle with 1 and ½ tablespoons of olive oil
7. Transfer the pulsed mixture to a serving dish and sprinkle with the basil
8. Serve and enjoy your delicious okra and tomato grilled side!

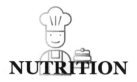

# NUTRITION

Kcal: 87.9

Fat: 7

Carbs: 5.8

Proteins: 2.6

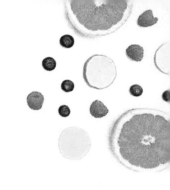

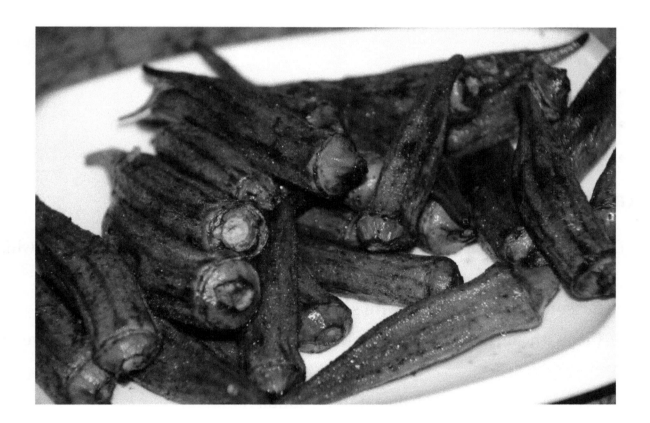

# Roasted Artichokes

Prep Time: 10 minutes| Cooking Time: 25 Minutes| Servings: 4

## INGREDIENTS:

- 5 Large artichokes
- ½ Medium pineapple, peeled and sliced into rounds
- 1 Medium lemon, juiced
- 2 tsp vinegar
- ½ Cup olive oil
- 1 Pinch salt
- 1 Pinch pepper

## DIRECTIONS:

1. Mix all together the vinegar with the lemon juice and olive oil and whisk very well
2. Season your ingredients with salt to taste
3. Clean the artichokes trim and cut into half; make sure to remove the chokes
4. Peel the pineapple and slice it into rounds
5. Bring a large pan of water to a boil with a steaming basket
6. When the water starts to boil, add the artichokes to the steamer and steam for about 25 minutes
7. Remove the artichokes from the water and drain; then brush it with the a little quantity of the prepared vinaigrette and transfer set aside

8. Heat a grill to a medium high heat and arrange the artichokes and the pineapple rings directly on the grill and grill for about 15 minutes over a medium heat

9. Remove your ingredients from the grill and transfer to a serving dish

10. Drizzle with the lemon vinaigrette; then serve and enjoy your delicious side!

**NUTRITION**

Kcal: 119.3

Fat: 4.1

Carbs: 12

Proteins: 6

# Roasted Red Peppers

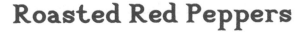

Prep Time: 10 minutes| Cooking Time: 45 Minutes| Servings: 4

## INGREDIENTS:

- 4 to 5 whole yellow and red peppers
- 1 Thinly sliced red onion
- 1 Teaspoon of mustard seeds
- 1 Finely diced garlic clove
- 2/3 Teaspoon of sea salt
- ½ Teaspoon of black pepper
- ½ Teaspoon of coriander seeds
- 2 Tablespoons of red wine vinegar
- 2 Tablespoons of olive oil

## DIRECTIONS:

1. Preheat your oven to a temperature of about 390 °F.
2. Toss the red peppers into a little bit of oil
3. Arrange the peppers into a baking tray lined with a foil
4. Place the tray into the oven close to the oven's grill
5. Roast the peppers for about 45 minutes; meanwhile; mix the sliced onions with the remaining ingredients and set it aside
6. Remove the cooked peppers from the oven and let it cool for about 20 minutes
7. Peel the skin of the peppers and slice it with a scissors into pieces
8. Make sure to remove the core of the peppers
9. Toss the peppers with the onions and top with olives and parsley

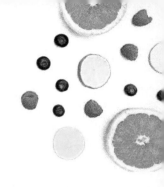

**10.** Serve and enjoy your appetizer!

## NUTRITION

Kcal: 106.5

Fat: 2.2

Carbs: 14

Proteins: 3

# Stuffed Zucchini

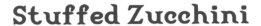

Prep Time: 15 minutes| Cooking Time: 25 Minutes| Servings: 6-7

## INGREDIENTS

- 6 to 7 medium zucchinis
- ½ Medium, diced brown onion
- 2 Tablespoons of pine nuts
- 7 Kalamata olives, without its pits
- 1 Small, chopped red chili
- 2 Peeled and roughly cut garlic cloves
- 1 Teaspoon of sweet paprika
- 2 Tablespoons of olive oil
- ½ Teaspoon of sea salt
- To make the Romesco Sauce
- ½ Large, seeded and cut red bell pepper
- 1 Small peeled and cut brown onion
- 1 Cup of zucchini flesh
- 1 to 2 garlic cloves
- 1 Teaspoon of apple cider vinegar
- 2 Tablespoon of tomato paste
- 1 Cup of water
- 2 Tablespoons of olive oil

## DIRECTIONS:

1. Carefully scoop out the flesh of the zucchini with a knife
2. Heat your oven to a temperature of about 360° F

3. Slice the zucchinis into half; then use a teaspoon to scoop out the flesh.

4. Chop about 1 cup of zucchini flesh and set it aside

5. Toast the pine nuts into a frying pan for about 1 minute

6. In the same pan; sauté the onion and the chili for about 1 minute; then sprinkle the paprika and sauté over a low heat

7. Process the garlic and the olives into a food processor

8. Mix the pine nuts, the sautéed onion and 1 pinch of salt and stir

9. Stuff the zucchinis with your fingers

10. Arrange the stuffed zucchinis over a baking tray greased with olive oil; then bake it into the oven for about 20 minutes at a temperature of about 360° F

11. To prepare the Romesco sauce, preheat a large non-stick frying pan over a medium heat

12. Sauté the onion and the red peppers into 2 tablespoons of olive oil for about 2 minutes.

13. Add the zucchini and the garlic and cook for 1 additional minute.

14. Add the tomato paste, the vinegar and the water; then mix very well and cook for 2 additional minutes

15. Turn off the heat and transfer the sauce to a food processor

16. Puree your ingredients until it is completely grounded

17. Serve and enjoy your dish!

**NUTRITION**

Kcal: 236

Fat: 7.3

Carbs: 13

Proteins: 12.6

# Cauliflower Rice

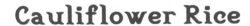

Prep Time: 5 minutes| Cooking Time: 10 Minutes| Servings: 6-7

## INGREDIENTS:

- 7 Oz Mushrooms, finely sliced
- 1 Medium cauliflower head, riced
- 1 Medium onion, finely minced
- 2 Cloves garlic, finely minced
- 1 ¼ Cups chicken stock
- 2 TBSP fresh parsley, finely minced
- 2 TBSP coconut oil, melted
- 1 Pinch salt
- 1 Pinch black pepper, freshly ground

## DIRECTIONS:

1. Heat the oil in a large skillet over a medium high heat
2. Add the onion and the garlic and sauté for about 2 minutes
3. Add in the mushrooms and sauté for about 2 minutes
4. Add the garlic and onion; cook until soft, about 1 to 2 minutes.
5. Add in the cauliflower rice, then cover and cook for about 5 minutes
6. Season with 1 pinch of salt and 1 pinch of pepper
7. Serve and enjoy your cauliflower risotto with topped with chopped fresh parsley!

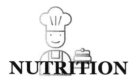

**NUTRITION**

Kcal: 119

Fat: 13.4

Carbs: 5

Proteins: 5

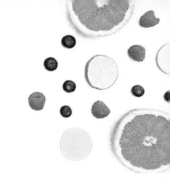

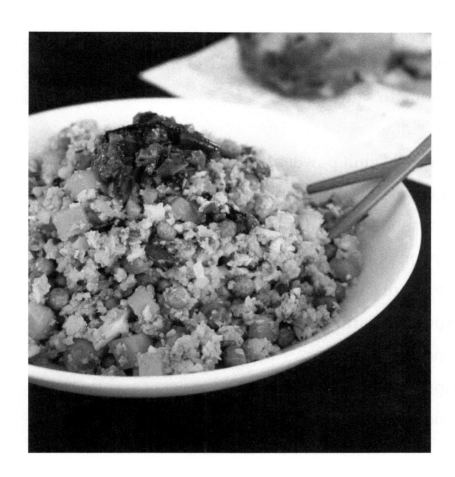

# Mushrooms caps with taco sauce

Prep Time: 10 minutes| Cooking Time: 10 Minutes| Servings: 5-6

## INGREDIENTS

- 3 to 4 large portabella mushroom caps with the stems and the gills removed
- ½ Cup of water

## INGREDDIENTS TO MAKE THE TACO SAUCE:

- 1 Can of tomato sauce
- ⅓ Cup of water
- ¼ Teaspoon of chili powder
- 1 and ½ teaspoons of cumin
- 1 and ½ teaspoons of minced onion
- 1 Tablespoon of white vinegar
- ½ Teaspoon of garlic powder
- ½ Teaspoon of garlic salt
- ¼ Teaspoon of paprika
- ¼ Teaspoon of honey
- ¼ Teaspoon of cayenne pepper

## DIRECTIONS

1. Place all the ingredients into a saucepan over a medium heat
2. Let the sauce simmer for about 15 minutes
3. Remove the saucepan from the heat and set it aside
4. Preheat your oven to a temperature of about 400° F.

5. Brush the sides of the mushrooms with a little bit of oil and season it with 1 pinch of salt and 1 pinch of pepper, add the minced onion, white vinegar; ½ Teaspoon of garlic powder, ½ Teaspoon of garlic salt, ¼ Teaspoon of paprika, ¼ Teaspoon of honey

6. Put the mushrooms over a foil lined with a baking sheet and bake it for about 10 minutes

7. Turn the mushrooms and bake it for about 4 to 6 minutes

8. Pour 1 tablespoon of the mushroom sauce over each of the mushrooms

9. Place the mushrooms back into the oven for about 4 to 5 minutes

10. Top with lettuce leaves and avocado slices

11. Serve and enjoy your dish!

## NUTRITION

Kcal: 109.5

Fat: 6.9

Carbs: 8.02

Proteins: 5.3.

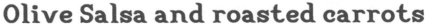

# Olive Salsa and roasted carrots

Prep Time: 10 minutes| Cooking Time: 25 Minutes| Servings: 5-6

**INGREDIENTS:**

- 1 Pound of carrots
- 2 Tablespoons of Olive oil
- 1 Tablespoon of honey
- ¼ Cup of water
- 1 Teaspoon of Salt
- To make the olive salsa
- To make the Olive Salsa
- 1 Cup of black unsalted and pitted olives
- 2 Teaspoons of drained and rinsed capers
- 1 Handful of finely chopped parsley
- 2 Tablespoons of finely chopped parsley
- 1 Tablespoon of Toasted pine nuts
- 3 Tablespoons of olive oil
- The juice of half a Lemon
- 1 Medium spring onion

**DIRECTIONS:**

1. Preheat your oven to a temperature of about 360°F
2. Line a baking sheet with a foil; then with a parchment paper
3. Peel the carrots and cut it into the form of quarters; then cut the quarters into halves in a lengthwise way
4. Transfer the carrots into a baking tray and drizzle it with olive oil
5. Add a little bit of honey and 1 pinch of salt

6. Pour about ¼ cup of water into your tray and cover it with a foil
7. Roast the carrots into the oven for about 25 minutes
8. Remove the tray from the oven and remove the foil; then place the carrots back into the oven and roast it for about 5 minutes
9. Remove the tray from the oven and place the carrots into a platter, then set it aside for about 5 minutes to cool
10. While you carrots are being roasted; make the salsa by finely chopping the olives; add the parsley and the spring onion
11. Add the capers; the lemon juice; the pine nuts and the Olive oil; then mix very well
12. When your carrots are cool; assemble it over a plate and spoon a little bit of salsa
13. Serve and enjoy your dinner!

## NUTRITION

Kcal: 109.1

Fat: 5.8

Carbs: 13

Proteins: 3

# Olive Salsa

Prep Time: 6 minutes| Cooking Time: 5 Minutes| Servings: 4

## INGREDIENTS:

- 1 Jar of pitted green olives
- 1 Can of pitted black olives
- 2 Garlic cloves
- 2 to 3 jalapeno chilies
- 1/3 Cup of Medium red onion
- 1 to 2 medium red peppers
- 1 to 2 Medium yellow peppers
- ½ Cup of toasted pine nuts
- 1 Tablespoon of chopped fresh parsley
- 2 Tablespoons of extra virgin olive oil
- 1 Tablespoon of red wine vinegar

## DIRECTIONS

1. To toast the pine nuts; heat it into a medium skillet over a low heat for about 5 minutes; make sure to stir very well
2. Drain the olives very well and chop it
3. Finely grate the garlic and remove the membranes of the jalapenos
4. Finely dice the onion and the red and the yellow peppers
5. Combine your ingredients in a bowl; then drizzle with olive oil and vinegar
6. Mix your ingredients very well and let it chill for about 6 hours
7. Serve and enjoy your olive salsa!

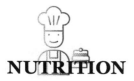

# NUTRITION

Kcal: 81

Fat: 8.2

Carbs: 3

Proteins: 4

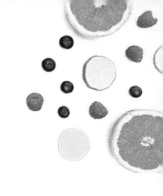

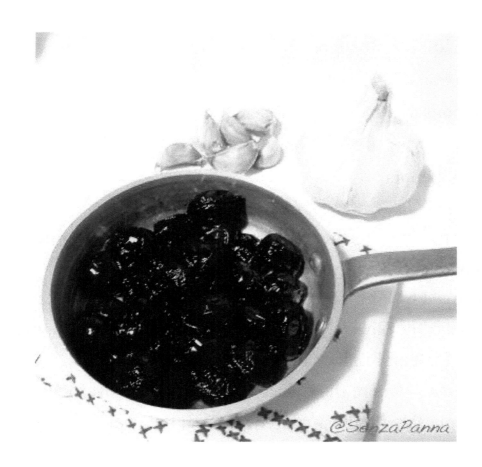

# Stuffed Squash

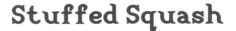

Prep Time: 10 minutes| Cooking Time: 20 Minutes| Servings: 4-5

## INGREDIENTS

- 1 Medium Kabocha squash, cut into halves with the seeds removed
- ¼ Diced red onion
- 1 Cup of diced zucchini
- ½ Cup of diced bell pepper
- 1 Tablespoon of extra virgin olive oil
- 2 Teaspoons of minced fresh rosemary
- 1 Pinch of salt
- 1 Pinch of pepper

## DIRECTIONS:

1. Preheat your oven to a temperature of about 350°F and line a baking sheet with a parchment paper.
2. Into a large bowl; mix altogether the chopped onion with the zucchini, the bell pepper; the olive oil and the fresh rosemary and season very well with 1 pinch of salt and 1 pinch of black pepper
3. Arrange the halves of the squash with the side-up over the baking sheet.
4. Fill the squash with the prepared stuffing; then bake it at a temperature of about 350°F for 20 minutes
5. Remove the stuffed squash from the oven; then serve and enjoy it warm!

## NUTRITION

Kcal: 107.98

Fat: 5.5

Carbs: 11.3

Proteins: 5.9

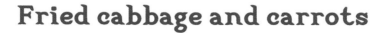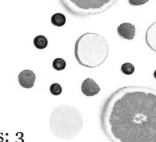

# Fried cabbage and carrots

Prep Time: 5 minutes| Cooking Time: 10 Minutes| Servings: 3

**INGREDIENTS:**

- 2 Pieces of 1 inch minced ginger
- 2 Minced garlic cloves
- 6 Cups of shredded cabbage
- 2 Cups of shredded carrots
- ½ Teaspoon of salt
- 2 Tablespoons of rice vinegar
- 2 Tablespoons of coconut aminos
- 4 Thinly sliced scallions
- 1 Tablespoon of toasted sesame oil
- Roasted black, sesame seeds
- Chopped cilantro

**DIRECTIONS:**

1. Place a wok over a medium heat and grease it with oil
2. When the oil heats up; add the ginger, the garlic and cook for about 30 seconds
3. Add the shredded cabbage, the carrots and the salt to the wok and sauté until your ingredients become tender for about 7 to 9 minutes
4. Add the coconut aminos; the rice vinegar, the scallions, and the sesame oil; then sauté for about 1 additional minute.
5. Top your dish with cilantro and black sesame seeds
6. Serve and enjoy your snack!

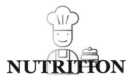

## NUTRITION

Kcal: 128.4

Fat: 3.2

Carbs: 16.5

Proteins: 4.6

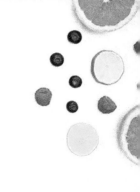

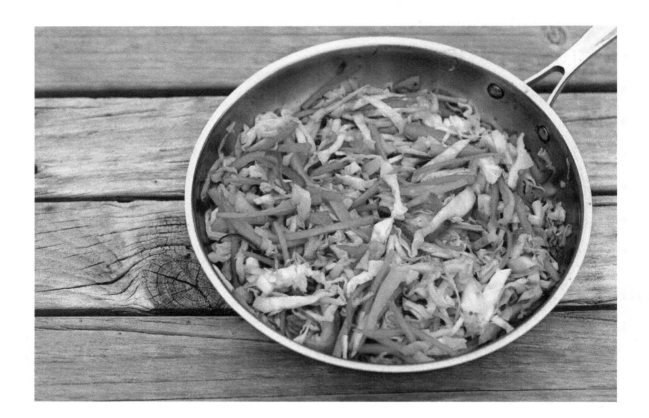

# RICE AND SUSHI RECIPES

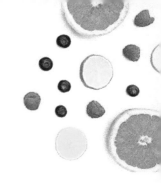

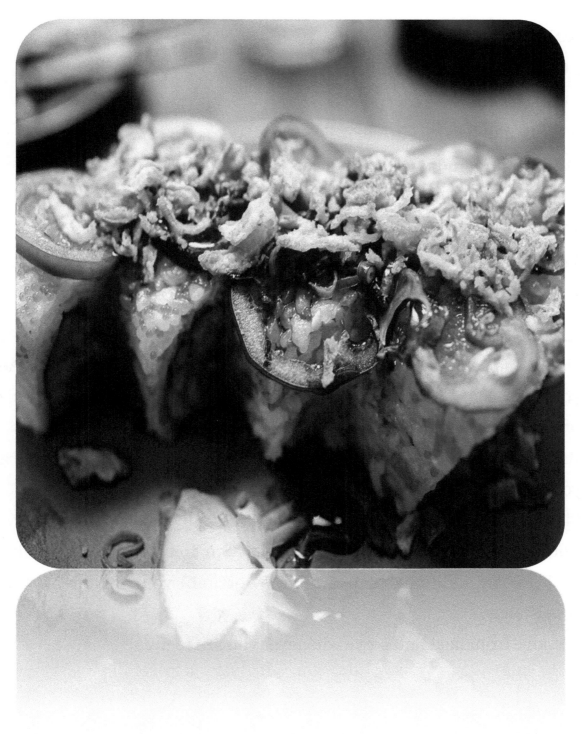

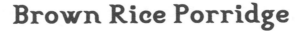

# Brown Rice Porridge

Prep Time: 10 minutes| Cooking Time: 20 Minutes| Servings: 3

## INGREDIENTS:

- 1 Cup of Brown Rice (Fully Cooked)
- 1 Cup of Milk (2% Low in Fat)
- 2 Tbsp. Blueberries (Dried or Fresh)
- Dash of Cinnamon (Ground Variety)
- 1 Tbsp. Honey (Raw)
- 1 Egg
- ¼ tsp. Vanilla
- 1 Tbsp. Butter

## DIRECTIONS:

1. Use a small - sized saucepan and place over medium to high heat. Add in your fully cooked brown rice, low-fat milk, dried or fresh blueberries, dash of ground cinnamon and raw honey. Stir thoroughly to combine.
2. Bring this mixture to a boil. Once boiling, reduce the heat to low and allow your mixture to simmer for the next 20 minutes.
3. Slowly drizzle in your beaten egg until thoroughly incorporate.
4. Add in your pure vanilla and soft butter. Stir to combine and continue to cook for an additional 1 to 2 minutes or until your mixture is thick in consistency.
5. Remove from heat and serve whenever you are ready.

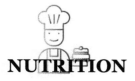

# NUTRITION

Kcal: 280

Fat: 6.7

Carbs: 70.1

Proteins: 14

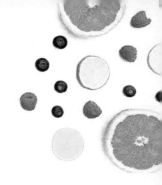

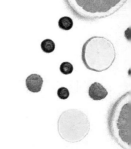

# Mushroom Rice

Prep Time: 10 minutes| Cooking Time: 45 Minutes| Servings: 3

## INGREDIENTS

- 3 cups of water
- 16 oz. mushrooms (sliced)
- 1 cup of almonds (slivered and blanched)
- 1 cup of brown rice
- 1/3 cup of pimientos (chopped)
- 3 tablespoons of butter
- 1 teaspoon of salt
- 1/8 teaspoon of black pepper

## DIRECTIONS:

1. In a medium saucepan, melt the butter over medium-high heat. Stir in the 16 ounces of sliced mushrooms and the 1 cup of slivered blanched almonds until they turn a golden brown.
2. Stir in the 3 cups of water
3. Add 1 cup of brown rice and 1/3 cup of chopped pimientos
4. Add 1 teaspoon of salt and 1/8 teaspoon of black pepper.
5. Turn heat to high and bring to a boil.
6. Reduce heat to low, cover, and simmer until the rice is tender for 45 additional minutes.
7. Serve warm!

# NUTRITION

Kcal: 233

Fat: 7.8

Carbs: 36

Proteins: 4.1

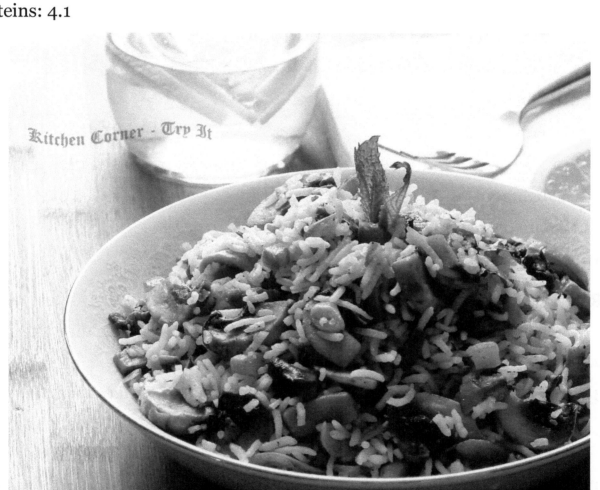

# Southern-Style Rice

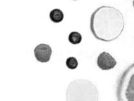

Prep Time: 8 minutes| Cooking Time: 15 Minutes| Servings: 3-4

## INGREDIENTS

- 2 and 1/2 cups of brown rice (cooked)
- 1 1/2 cups of chicken breast (cooked and cubed)
- 1 cup of black beans (cooked and drained, either canned or cooked from dried beans)
- 2/3 cup of salsa
- 1/2 cup of Monterey jack cheese (grated plus a little extra for garnishment), 1/2 cup of corn (canned),
- 1/2 cup of tomatoes (chopped fine)
- Sour cream for garnishment

## DIRECTIONS:

1. Cook the 2 1/2 cups of brown rice according to the package directions.
2. At the same time, cook the 1 1/2 cups of chicken.
3. Either boil the chicken for 20 minutes in a pot of water, or grill it in the oven until done, or pan fry it until done for about 10-20 minutes, depending on how big the chicken breast is.
4. Next, place the hot cooked rice and hot cubed chicken in a medium saucepan, add the 1 cup of black beans, 2/3 cup of salsa, 1/2 cup of canned corn, 1/2 cup of chopped tomatoes, and warm over medium-low heat constantly stirring for about 15 minutes.
5. Remove from heat and put into a serving dish.
6. Toss in the 1/2 cup of Monterey jack cheese, tossing to melt the cheese.

7. Garnish the top with extra grated Monterey jack cheese and a couple dollops of sour cream.

8. Alternately, you can dollop the sour cream on individual portions

**NUTRITION**

Kcal: 178.4

Fat: 2.9

Carbs: 23

Proteins: 15.5

# Ginger Rice

Prep Time: 10 minutes| Cooking Time: 10 Minutes| Servings: 3

## INGREDIENTS

- 6 cups of water
- 3 cups of brown rice (long grain)
- 1 teaspoon of salt
- 1/2 teaspoon of ginger (ground)

## DIRECTIONS:

1. Place a large pot on medium heat and pour in the 6 cups of water, 3 cups of long grain brown rice, 1 teaspoon of salt, and 1/2 teaspoon of ground ginger.

2. Bring the liquid to a boil, stir, and then cover tight after reducing the heat to simmer.

3. Do not lift the lid or stir during this part, just allow the rice to cook untouched; this helps each grain to absorb the liquid and be tender. If the rice is disturbed during this, the result is grains that may not be tender.

4. Simmer for 50 minutes. Completely take off heat and have it stand for an additional 10 minutes, and be sure to keep the lid on the pot. Fluff with a fork, pour into a serving bowl and serve.

## NUTRITION

Kcal: 161.6

Fat: 3.9

Carbs: 28.7

Proteins: 3.8

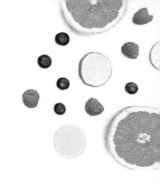

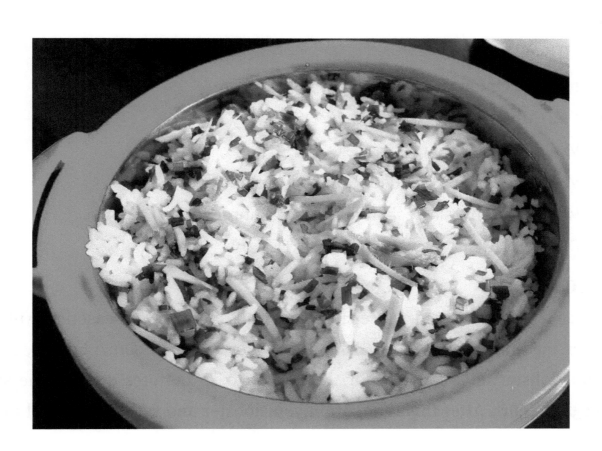

# Lobster Risotto

Prep Time: 10 minutes| Cooking Time: 20 Minutes| Servings: 3

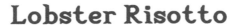

## INGREDIENTS:

- 1 lb of Lobster Tails (Frozen and Thawed)
- 4 ½ Cups of Chicken Stock
- 4 Tbsp. of Butter
- 1 Cup of Onion (Finely Chopped)
- 1 ½ Cups of Brown rice
- ½ Cup of Brandy
- ½ Cup of Parmesan Cheese (Freshly Grated)
- ¼ Cup of Chives (Fresh and Roughly Chopped)
- Dash of Salt and Black Pepper(For Taste)

## DIRECTIONS:

1. Place a medium sized saucepan filled with some water seasoned with salt over medium to high heat. Bring this water to a boil. Once boiling, add in your lobster tails and boil for the next 8 to 10 minutes or until the shells begin to curl. After this time, drain your lobster and set aside to cool for the next 15 minutes.

2. After this time, remove the lobster meat from the shells and cut into small sized pieces. Set aside for later use.

3. Then use a medium sized saucepan. Set over medium heat and add in your homemade chicken stock. Bring this stock to a boil. Reduce the heat to low.

4. Using a large-sized saucepan, place it over medium heat. Add in your butter and once your butter is fully melted, continue to cook for at least 1 to 1 ½ minutes or until your butter begins to turn brown in color.

5. Add in your rice and stir thoroughly to coat in your brown butter. Add your brandy and allow to simmer for the next 3 minutes or until the liquid has been fully evaporated. Then add in at least half a cup of your stock and stir to combine. Continue to cook for another 2 minutes.

6. Continue to cook your rice for the next 20 minutes or until your rice is tender to the touch. Once tender remove from heat

7. Add in your grated Parmesan cheese, remaining butter and at least two spoonfuls of your chives. Season your mixture with a dash of salt and black pepper. Stir thoroughly to combine.

8. Transfer your freshly made risotto into a large sized serving dish. Place your lobster tail on top and garnish with your remaining chives. Serve whenever you are ready.

**NUTRITION**

Kcal: 562

Fat: 19.3

Carbs: 58.2

Proteins: 23.6

# Rice with Cornish Hens

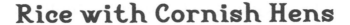

Prep Time: 10 minutes| Cooking Time: 50 Minutes| Servings: 4

## INGREDIENTS

- 4 Cornish Style Hens (Giblets Removed and Toss Out)
- Dash of Salt and Black Pepper (For Taste)
- 2 tsp. of Olive Oil
- ½ Cup of Scallions (Minced)
- 1 tsp. of Thyme (Dried)
- 1 Cup of Brown Rice
- 1 ½ Cups of Chicken Broth (Evenly Divided)
- 1 Cup of Tomatoes (Finely Chopped)
- 1 Bell Pepper (Green in Color and Finely Chopped)
- Some Cranberry Sauce (optional).

## DIRECTIONS:

1. The first thing that you will want to do is preheat your oven to 450 degrees.

2. While your oven is heating up; rinse your Cornish thoroughly, Pat dry with a few paper towels and season with a generous amount of salt and pepper. Place your hens into a large sized baking pan and set aside for later use.

3. Heat up a large sized saucepan placed over medium heat. Add in some oil and once your oil is hot enough add in your garlic and scallions. Cook for the next 2 minutes before adding in your rice and thyme. Stir thoroughly to combine.

4. Add in your homemade chicken broth and cover. Allow your rice to cook at a simmer for at least 3 minutes before adding in your chopped tomatoes and chopped green bell pepper. Season with a dash of salt and pepper

5. Remove from heat and place your rice mixture into the inside of your hens. Pour your remaining homemade chicken broth into your large sized roasting pan with your hens.

6. Place into your oven. Reduce the heat of your oven to bake at 350 degrees. Bake for at least 50 minutes to an hour or until your hens are fully cooked through. Make sure to baste your hens every 10 minutes with the juices in your roasting pan.

7. Remove from your oven and allow standing for at least 10 minutes. Carve and serve with your pan juices poured over the top.

**NUTRITION**

Kcal: 400

Fat: 15.5

Carbs: 12.3

Proteins: 50.1

# Pecan Brown Rice

Prep Time: 10 minutes| Cooking Time: 55 Minutes| Servings: 3-4

## INGREDIENTS

- 4 cups of water
- 3 cups of brown rice
- 2 cups of beef broth
- 1 1/2 cups of pecans (toasted)
- 4 stalks of celery (chopped)
- 2 green onions (chopped greens and all)
- 1 tablespoon of Worcestershire sauce
- 1 tablespoon of butter,
- salt and black pepper to season

## DIRECTIONS:

1. In a large saucepan, pour the 4 cups of water, 2 cups of beef broth, and 1 tablespoon of Worcestershire sauce, stir together, and bring the mixture to a boil over high heat.

2. Stir in the 3 cups of brown rice after the liquid begins to boil. Turn to low heat once the rice is added, cover and cook until the rice is tender for about an additional 40 minutes, check the rice to see and when tender, turn off the heat.

3. Meanwhile, melt the 1 tablespoon of butter in a large skillet and sauté the chopped celery and chopped onions, until tender.

4. Stir in the 1 1/2 cups of toasted pecans.

5. Once the rice is cooked, pour it in and stir.

6. Season the rice with the salt and black pepper to taste. Serve immediately.

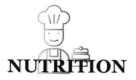

# NUTRITION

Kcal: 212.6

Fat: 6.7

Carbs: 32.8

Proteins: 5.1

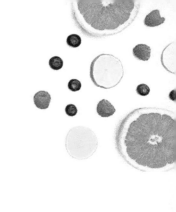

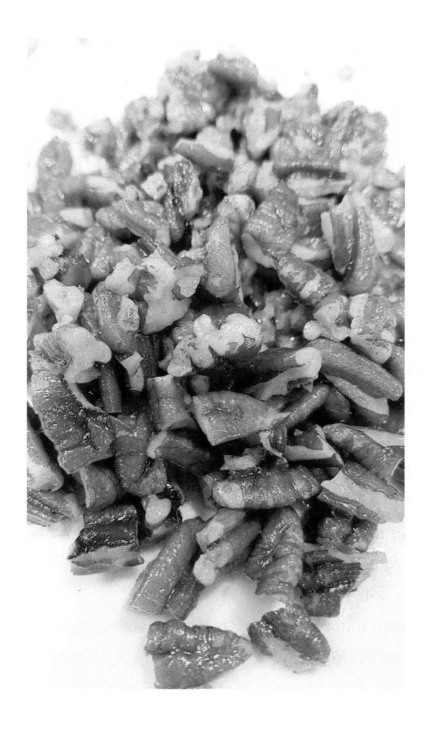

# Lemon rice with cheese

Prep Time: 10 minutes| Cooking Time: 1 ½ Hours| Servings: 4

## INGREDIENTS

- 2 1/2 cups of chicken broth
- 1 1/2 cups of brown rice
- 1 onion (chopped fine)
- 1 lemon (juice and zest only)
- 1/2 cup of Parmesan cheese (grated)
- 1/4 cup of parsley (minced fresh)
- 1/4 cup of basil (minced fresh)
- 1 tablespoon of olive oil
- 1/2 teaspoon of salt
- 1/4 teaspoon of black pepper

## DIRECTIONS:

1. Place oven rack in the middle and preheat to 375 degrees Fahrenheit.
2. In an 8x8 baking dish, spread the 1 1/2 cups of rice.
3. In a medium-sized saucepan over medium-low heat, add the tablespoon of olive oil, and then stir in the finely chopped onion for about 10 minutes.
4. Add the 2 1/2 cups of chicken broth to the onions and turn the heat to high to bring to a boil.
5. Once the broth and onions boil, remove from heat, and carefully pour over the rice in the baking dish.
6. Cover the rice air tight with aluminum foil and bake for an hour or longer until the rice tenderizes.
7. Once rice is tender, remove from oven and take a fork to fluff the rice.

8. Stir in the lemon juice / zest, 1/2 cup of Parmesan cheese, 1/4 cup of fresh minced parsley, 1/4 cup of fresh minced basil, and the salt and black pepper.

9. Cover loosely with the foil and allow sitting for another 5 minutes before serving.

**NUTRITION**

Kcal: 220.4

Fat: 8.3

Carbs: 17.

Proteins: 20.6

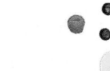

# Rice Balls

Prep Time: 10 minutes| Cooking Time: 25 Minutes| Servings: 4-5

**INGREDIENTS:**

- 1 1/4 pounds of Swiss chard leaves
- 1 jar of marinara sauce (26 ounce)
- 2 cups of brown rice (short grain cooked)
- 1 cup of arugula leaves (chopped and packed)
- 1 cup of cream cheese (softened 8 ounce package)
- 1 cup of lentils (cooked)
- 1/2 cup of mint leaves (chopped)
- 1/2 cup of Parmesan (grated)
- 1/4 cup of olive oil
- 2 garlic cloves (minced)
- 2 tablespoons of butter
- 1 teaspoon of salt
- 1/2 teaspoon of black pepper
- dash of salt and cooking spray

**DIRECTIONS:**

1. Ahead of time, cook the 2 cups of short grain brown rice and the 1 cup of lentils according to the package directions.
2. Preheat the oven to 400 degrees Fahrenheit, and place the rack in the center.
3. Spray a 9x13 baking dish with cooking spray.
4. Meanwhile, take the Swiss chard leaves and pull the stems off. Half each leaf lengthwise

5. Add water to a large pot and bring it to a boil then add the dash of salt and the Swiss chard leaves and boil for a short 10 seconds.

6. Immediately remove the chard leaves and gently rinse in cold water. Dry on a paper towel.

7. In a separate bowl, stir in the 2 cups of cooked brown rice, 1 cup of cooked lentils, 1 cup of arugula leaves, 1 cup of softened cream cheese, 1/2 cup of chopped mint leaves, 1/4 cup of olive oil, 2 cloves of minced garlic, and the 1/2 teaspoon of pepper. Spoon the rice mixture (about 1/3 cup) into the chard leaves, one at a time, rolling the leaves into a "roll."

8. Pour about a cup of the marinara sauce into the baking dish over the cooking spray.

9. Carefully add the chard rolls, making sure they do not unroll, all on the bottom of the baking dish.

10. Pour the remaining marinara sauce over the top; then dust with the 1/2 cup of parmesan cheese.

11. Chop the 2 tablespoons of butter and sprinkle them on top.
    Bake in the oven for 25 minutes. Allow to cool for 10 minutes prior to serving.

## NUTRITION

Kcal: 116.3

Fat: 1.7

Carbs: 18.5

Proteins: 5.8

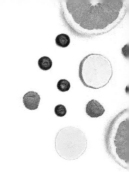
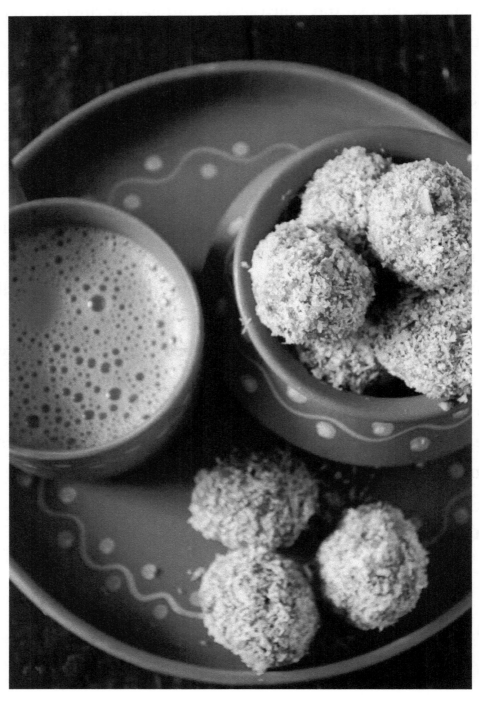

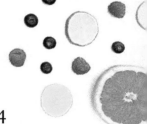

# Chickpea and rice casserole

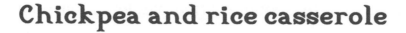

Prep Time: 10 minutes| Cooking Time: 45 Minutes| Servings: 4

## INGREDIENTS:

- 3 1/2 cups of brown rice (cooked)
- 2 cans of chickpeas (15 Oz each, drained)
- 1 can of tomatoes (28 Oz undrained)
- 1 onion (chopped)
- 3 tablespoons of tahini
- 3 tablespoons of water
- 1 tablespoon of sesame seeds (toasted)
- 1 1/2 teaspoon of parsley (dried)
- 1 teaspoon of garlic powder
- 1 teaspoon of oregano (dried)
- 1 teaspoon of basil (dried)
- Salt and black pepper to season

## DIRECTIONS:

1. Cook the 3 1/2 cups of brown rice according to package directions (to make 3 1/2 cups of cooked rice).

2. In a separate cup, stir the 3 tablespoons of tahini with the 3 tablespoons of water till well combined and set it aside.

3. Preheat the oven to 375 degrees Fahrenheit.

4. Spray a 9x13 pan with cooking spray.

5. Add the 3 1/2 cups of cooked rice into the 9x13 pan and stir in the 2 cans of chickpeas, 1 can of tomatoes, chopped onion, a tablespoon of toasted

sesame seeds, 1 1/2 teaspoon of dried parsley, 1 teaspoon of garlic powder, 1 teaspoon of dried oregano, and the 1 teaspoon of dried basil.

6. Season with the salt and black pepper and stir together.

7. Stir in the tahini and water mixture, making sure it spreads throughout.

8. Place in the center of the oven and bake until the top turns a golden brown, for about 40 minutes.

9. Remove from oven, sprinkle the sesame seeds over the top and return to oven to bake for another 5 minutes.

10. Cool for up to 10 minutes and serve immediately.

## NUTRITION

Kcal: 116.3

Fat: 1.7

Carbs: 18.5

Proteins: 5.8

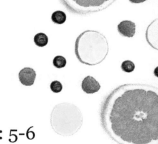

# Rice with cashew

Prep Time: 10 minutes| Cooking Time: 15 Minutes| Servings: 5-6

**INGREDIENTS:**

- 2 pounds of chicken (cut breasts - boneless and skinless)
- 4 cups of chicken broth
- 2 cups of brown rice (cooked)
- 1 red bell pepper (thinly sliced and seeded)
- 10 water chestnut
- 1 cup of green peas (frozen)
- 1 cup of cashews (raw)
- 3/4 cup of onion (thinly sliced)
- 1/2 cup of onion (chopped)
- 1/4 cup of maple syrup
- 4 garlic cloves (chopped)
- 2 1/2 tablespoons of soy sauce
- 2 1/2 tablespoons of honey
- 2 1/2 tablespoons of parsley leaves (chopped)
- 2 tablespoons of butter (divided)
- 2 tablespoons of canola oil
- 2 tablespoons of grill seasoning
- 1 1/2 tablespoons of ground chipotle powder
- 1 tablespoon of ground cumin
- 1 tablespoon of olive oil

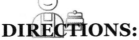
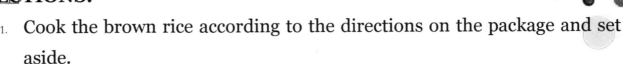

## DIRECTIONS:

1. Cook the brown rice according to the directions on the package and set aside.

2. Heat a mid-sized pot over medium heat and add the 1 tablespoon of olive oil and 1 tablespoon of butter.

3. Once the butter melts, stir in the 1/2 cup of chopped onion and sauté a couple of minutes.

4. Stir in the cooked rice and heat for a couple of minutes.

5. Pour the 4 cups of chicken broth over the rice and turn heat to high to bring the liquid to a boil.

6. Then reduce heat to simmer for about 10 minutes.

7. Meanwhile, pour the 2 tablespoons of canola oil into a hot skillet and add the chicken, keeping the heat on high.

8. Sprinkle with the 2 tablespoons of grill seasoning, completely brown the chicken.

9. At the last minute, add the 2 1/2 tablespoons of soy sauce and stir in the 3/4 cup of sliced onions, chopped bell pepper, and the garlic cloves.

10. Stir and cook for 3 minutes, stir in the cup of green peas, the water chestnuts and the cashews and heat through.

11. Stir in the 1 tablespoon of ground cumin and the 1 1/2 tablespoons of chipotle powder.

12. Coat with the honey and maple syrup, turn the heat off, and then toss the 2 1/2 tablespoons of parsley.

13. To serve, spoon rice onto a plate and top with the chicken mixture.

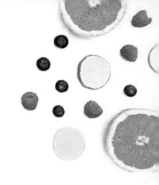

## NUTRITION

Kcal: 282.5

Fat: 21

Carbs: 20.1

Proteins: 6.5

# KETOGENIC RECIPES

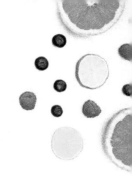

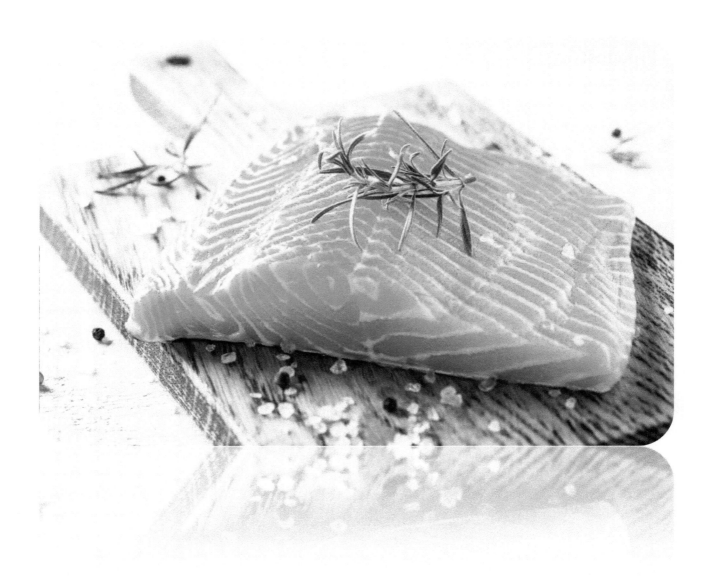

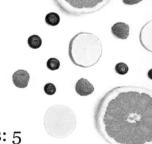

# Eggplant Cannelloni

Prep Time: 15 minutes| Cooking Time: 20 Minutes| Servings: 5

## INGREDIENTS

- To make the Basil and the Spinach Filling
- 2 Cups of soaked cashews
- 3 Crushed garlic cloves
- ¼ Cup of nutritional yeast
- 1 Tablespoon of lemon juice
- ½ Cup of almond milk
- ½ Cup of basil
- ¾ cup of spinach
- ¼ Teaspoon of salt
- ½ Teaspoon of pepper
- 2 Eggplants
- To make the tomato Sauce
- 2 Tablespoons of olive oil
- 2 Minced garlic cloves
- 1 Can of chopped tomatoes
- 1 Teaspoon of honey
- 1 Pinch of salt
- 1Pinch of pepper
- 2 Tablespoons of chopped basil

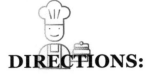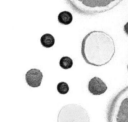

## DIRECTIONS:

1. Preheat your oven to a temperature of about 350° F

2. Drain the cashews; then place it into a food processor with the nutritional yeast

3. Add the lemon juice and the almond milk; then blend it until you obtain a creamy mixture

4. Add the spinach and the basil; then pulse it very well

5. Season the spinach with 1 pinch of salt and 1 pinch of pepper; then set it aside

6. Slice the eggplants with clean paper towels in order to remove any excess of salt

7. Bake the eggplant in the oven for about 15 minutes at a temperature of about 390° F

8. Make the sauce by heating the olive oil into a saucepan over a medium heat; then add the garlic and let cook for about 10 minutes

9. Season very well with 1 pinch of salt, 1 pinch of pepper

10. Pour a small quantity of the sauce into the bottom of a baking tray

11. Put around 2 to 3 spoonfuls of the basil mixture and the spinach over the slices of the eggplants

12. Tightly roll the eggplant slices and place it into the baking tray

13. Pour the remaining quantity of the sauce over the eggplants and bake it for about 15 minutes

14. Remove the eggplant cannelloni from the oven and top it with chopped basil

15. Serve and enjoy your lunch!

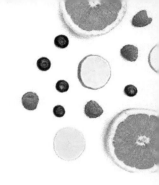

## NUTRITION

Kcal: 226.7

Fat: 10.2

Carbs: 16

Proteins: 17

# Zucchini Lasagna

Prep Time: 10 minutes| Cooking Time: 20 Minutes| Servings: 4

## INGREDIENTS

- To make the Basil-Cashew Cheese:
- 1 Cup of unsalted cashews
- ½ cup unsweetened almond milk
- ¼ Cup of fresh basil leaves
- 2 Minced garlic cloves
- ½ Teaspoon of sea salt
- To make the Artichoke-Tomato Sauce
- 1 Tablespoon of olive oil
- 1 Diced onion
- 2 Minced garlic cloves
- 1 can of unsalted diced tomatoes, about 1 and ½ cups
- 1 Can of 8 ounces of unsalted tomato sauce
- 1 Cup of chopped marinated artichoke hearts
- ¼ Cup of fresh basil leaves
- Pepper flakes
- 1 Pinch of sea salt
- 1 Pinch of Freshly-ground black pepper
- To make the Zucchini Lasagne
- 5 or 6 medium zucchinis
- 1 Pinch of coarse salt

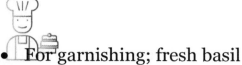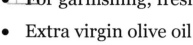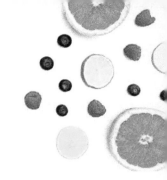

- For garnishing; fresh basil
- Extra virgin olive oil

## DIRECTIONS:

1. To make the basil-cashew Cheese
2. Start by soaking the cashews into a bowl filled with water and set it aside for about 30 minutes.
3. Drain the cashews and rinse it very well; then add your ingredients into a food processor or a blender and process it until it becomes smooth
4. To make the artichoke-Tomato Sauce; heat the oil into a large non-stick skillet
5. Add the diced onions and sauté it for about 3 minutes
6. Add the garlic and cook it for about 2 minutes
7. Add the tomato sauce, the diced tomatoes and the artichoke hearts
8. Add the basil leaves and toss in the basil leaves
9. Season with 1 pinch of sea salt and let the sauce boil over a low heat for about 10 minutes
10. To make the zucchini Lasagna
11. Preheat your oven to a temperature of about 375° F
12. Slice the zucchini into thick slices
13. Season the zucchini and set it aside for about 20 minutes and drain as much water as you can
14. Grease a baking tray with olive oil; then lay the zucchini slices into the bottom
15. Top the zucchini slices with about ½ cup of the sauce and about ¼ cup of cashew cheese.

16. Repeat the same process with the rest of the ingredients; then garnish it with fresh basil

17. Drizzle with olive oil and bake your lasagna for about 20 minutes

18. Set the lasagna aside for about 15 minutes

19. Serve and enjoy your lasagna!

**NUTRITION**

Kcal: 182.3

Fat: 7.4

Carbs: 15

Proteins: 10.5

# Green salad dressing

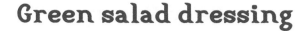
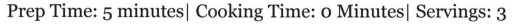

Prep Time: 5 minutes| Cooking Time: 0 Minutes| Servings: 3

**INGREDIENTS:**

**For the Dressing:**

- ½ Cup of extra virgin olive oil
- ½ Cup of apple cider vinegar
- 1 Medium lemon, the juice only
- 1 and ½ teaspoons of garlic powder
- 1 and ½ teaspoons of dried oregano
- 1 and ½ teaspoons of dried basil
- 1 Teaspoon of parsley
- 1 Teaspoon of mustard
- ½ Teaspoon of onion powder
- 1 Pinch of salt
- 1 Pinch of pepper
- 1 Pinch of pepper

**DIRECTIONS:**

1. Whisk all your ingredients all together
2. Pour into the dressing bottle
3. Serve over your favourite Greek Salad
4. Enjoy your salad with the dressing!

**NUTRITION**

Kcal: 150
Fat: 17
Carbs: 1
Proteins: 0.5

# Beef Gravy

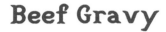

Prep Time:10 minutes| Cooking Time: 10 Minutes| Servings: 3

## INGREDIENTS:

- 2 Tablespoons of Whole Egg Mayonnaise
- 2 Tablespoons of small finely chopped gherkin
- ¼ Teaspoon of white vinegar
- ¼ Teaspoon of garlic powder
- ¼ Teaspoon of onion powder
- ½ Teaspoon of mustard powder
- 1Teaspoon of finely chopped dill finely
- ¼ Teaspoon of sweet paprika
- 1 Pinch of white ground pepper
- 1 Teaspoon of erythritol

## DIRECTONS:

1. In a small mixing bowl, add the whole egg mayonnaise, the finely chopped gherkin, the garlic powder, the onion powder, the mustard powder, the finely chopped dill, the sweet paprika and the white ground pepper and mix very well
2. Store in the refrigerator for an overnight
3. Serve and enjoy your dipping sauce with chicken wings!

## NUTRITION

Kcal: 351.3

Fat: 34.7

Carbs: 2.5

Proteins: 10.1

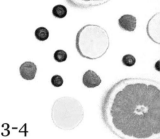

# Ketogenic Dressing

Prep Time: 5 minutes| Cooking Time: 0 Minutes| Servings: 3-4

## INGREDIENTS:

- 1/3 Cup of Low Carb Mayonnaise
- 1 Tablespoon of sour cream
- ½ Tablespoon of sugar-free tomato sauce
- 1 Teaspoons Frank's hot sauce
- ½ Teaspoon of dried minced onion
- ½ Teaspoon of lemon juice
- 1 Teaspoon of finely grated horseradish
- ¼ Teaspoon of garlic powder
- 1 Pinch of salt
- 1 Pinch of pepper

## DIRECTIONS:

1. In a small bowl; add all the low carb Mayonnaise with the sour cream, the tomato sauce, the Frank's hot sauce, the dried minced onion, the lemon juice, the finely grated horseradish, the garlic powder, the salt and the pepper
2. Whisk your ingredients very well
3. Place into the fridge and let marinate for about 1 hour
4. Use your Keto dressing or you can also use it as a dip!

## NUTRITION

Kcal: 44
Fat: 4.8
Carbs: 1.6
Proteins: 0.38

# Cheese sauce

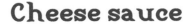
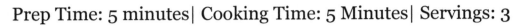

Prep Time: 5 minutes| Cooking Time: 5 Minutes| Servings: 3

## INGREDIENTS:

- 1.6 Ounces of Cream Cheese
- 1/8 Cup of Butter
- 1 Tablespoon of Heavy Cream
- 1 Tablespoon of mozzarella cheese

## DIRECTONS:

1. In a saucepan, place the cream cheese, the butter and the heavy cream; then place over a low heat.
2. Keep stirring until the cheese melts and all your ingredients are very well combined
3. Add in the mozzarella cheese; then whisk very well
4. You can use the sauce immediately or store in the refrigerator

## NUTRITION

Kcal: 389

Fat: 39

Carbs: 2

Proteins: 6

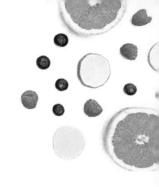

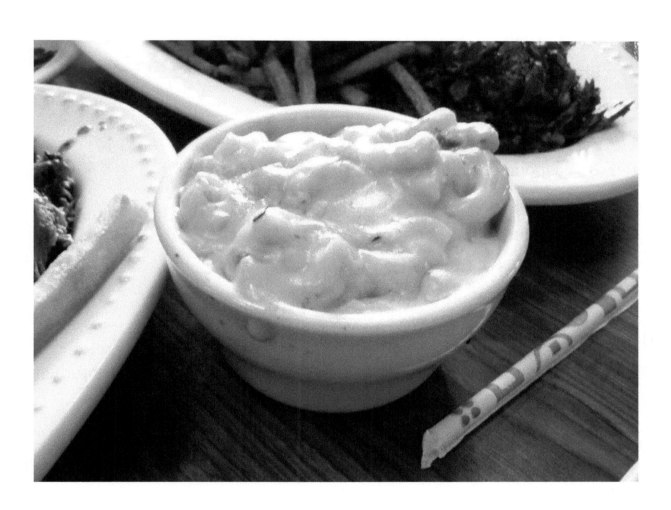

# Keto Guacamole

Prep Time: 5 minutes| Cooking Time: 0 Minutes| Servings: 3

## INGREDIENTS:

- 1 Medium Avocado
- 1 Teaspoon of Lime Juice
- 1 Pinch of salt
- 2 Pinches of pepper
- ¼ Teaspoon of Cumin
- 1 Garlic clove
- 1/8 Teaspoon of Chilli Powder
- 1/8 teaspoon of Smoked Paprika
- 1 Tablespoon of finely chopped Cilantro
- 2 Tablespoons of thinly sliced scallions
- 1 Tablespoon of Sour Cream

## DIRECTIONS:

1. Start by splitting the avocados; then remove the seeds and scoop the flesh in a bowl; then add in the lime juice
2. Mash the avocado with a fork
3. Add in the rest of the ingredients and mix very well
4. Serve with low carb flaxseed crackers!

## NUTRITION

Kcal: 115

Fat: 10

Carbs: 7

Proteins: 7

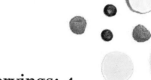

# Chimichurri Sauce

Prep Time: 10 minutes| Cooking Time: 0 Minutes| Servings: 4

## INGREDIENTS:

- 1 Tablespoon of parsley
- 1 Garlic clove
- ½ Small red chili; with the seeds removed
- ¼ Tablespoon of oregano leaves
- ¼ Tablespoon of red wine vinegar
- 1 Tablespoon of olive oil
- 1 Pinch of salt
- 1 Pinch of black pepper

## DIRECTIONS:

1. Start by cutting the chillies down the middle; then deseed them
2. Finely chop the parsley, the chili, and the oregano
3. Crush the garlic; then add to a bowl with the vinegar, the oil, the salt and the pepper
4. Mix your ingredients very well with a spoon; then set aside for about 30 minutes
5. Serve or store in the refrigerator
6. Enjoy!

## NUTRITION

Kcal: 76

Fat: 8.2

Carbs: 0.7

Proteins: 0.2

# Mushroom sauce

Prep Time: 7 minutes| Cooking Time: 20 Minutes| Servings: 3-4

## INGREDIENTS:

- ½ Tablespoon of coconut oil, melted
- 1 Minced garlic clove
- ¼ Thinly sliced small onion
- 1 Pinch of salt
- 1 Pinch of ground black pepper
- 3.5 Ounces of mushrooms thinly sliced
- 2.5 Teaspoons of Worcestershire sauce
- ½ Tablespoon of Dijon mustard
- ¼ Cup of heavy cream
- 1 Tablespoons of finely chopped fresh tarragon

## DIRECTIONS:

1. Put a saucepan over a high heat; then add in the butter, the garlic, the onion, the salt, and the pepper and sauté until the onions start to turn translucent for about 2 minutes
2. Add in the mushrooms and sauté for about 3 minutes
3. Add in the Worcestershire sauce, the Dijon mustard, and the cream.
4. Let simmer for about 10 to 15 minutes or until the sauce starts thickening.
5. Add in the tarragon; then serve and enjoy!

## NUTRITION

Kcal: 165
Fat: 8
Carbs: 7
Proteins: 3

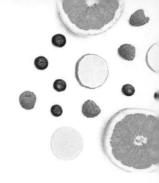

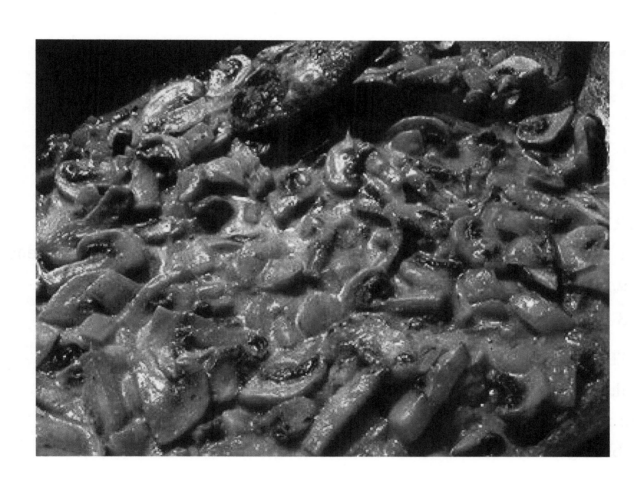

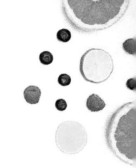

# Keto Mayonnaise

Prep Time: 5 minutes| Cooking Time: 20 Minutes| Servings: 4

## INGREDIENTS:

- ¼ Cup of olive oil
- 1 Egg
- ¼ Teaspoon of Mustard of your choice
- ½ Teaspoon of Vinegar or Lime Juice
- 1/8 Teaspoon of Black Pepper
- 1/8 Teaspoon of salt

## DIRECTIONS:

1. Blend your ingredients except for the oil with a food processor or a blender
2. Add in the oil in about 1/3rd at a time; then blend very well
3. Store in the refrigerator or just serve immediately!

## NUTRITION

Kcal: 95

Fat: 11

Carbs: 0.5

Proteins: 3

# SALAD RECIPES

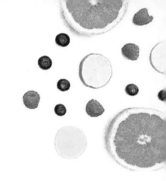

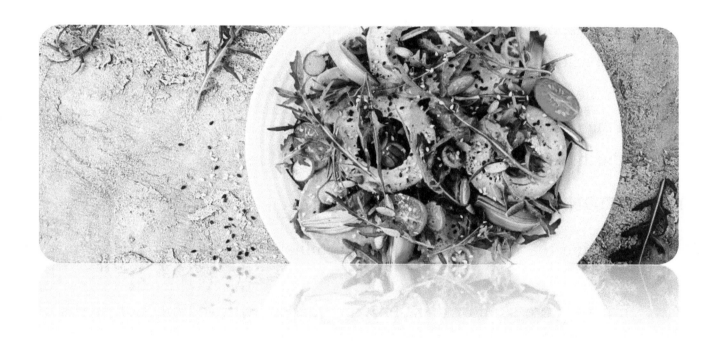

# Beet Salad

Prep Time: 5 minutes| Cooking Time: 0Minutes| Servings: 3

## INGREDIENTS:

- 2 Large beets, peeled, boiled and chopped
- 1 Small white onion, peeled and chopped
- 1 Medium ripe tomato, finely chopped
- 2 Tablespoons of olive oil
- 2 Tablespoons of fresh and finely chopped Chives and parsley
- 3 Tablespoons of olive oil
- 2 Tablespoons of balsamic vinegar
- 1 Pinch of salt
- 1 Pinch of freshly ground black pepper

## DIRECTIONS:

1. Combine the diced avocado, onion, tomato and beets in a large mixing bowl
2. In a separate shallow dish, mix the vinegar with the oil, salt, herbs and pepper
3. Dress your veggies with the vinegar and oil and toss very well
4. Refrigerate the salad for about 1 hour
5. Garnish with chopped chives and flat parsley
6. Serve and enjoy your salad!

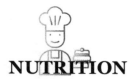

# NUTRITION

Kcal: 122.1

Fat: 7.9

Carbs: 9.8

Proteins: 3.7

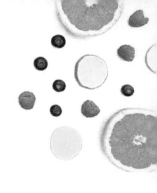

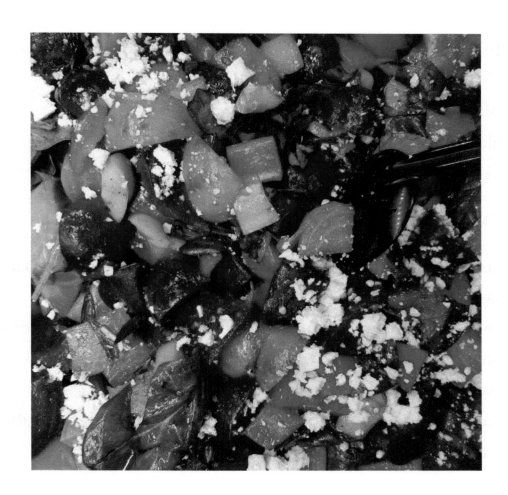

# Fruit Salad

Prep Time: 5 minutes| Cooking Time: 5 Minutes| Servings: 3

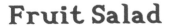

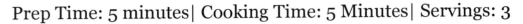

## INGREDIENTS

- 1 Pound of thinly sliced, hulled strawberries
- 3 Thinly sliced medium peaches
- 1 Cup of blueberries
- 1 Tablespoon of chopped fresh mint
- 2 Tablespoons of lemon juice
- 1 Tablespoon of honey
- 2 Teaspoons of balsamic vinegar

## DIRECTIONS:

1. In a serving bowl, mix the peaches, the strawberries, the blueberries and the basil.
2. Drizzle with the lemon juice, the maple syrup and the balsamic vinegar right on top.
3. Toss your ingredients gently to combine it very well
4. Immediately serve your fruit salad or let it chill in the refrigerator
5. Serve and enjoy your salad!

## NUTRITION

Kcal: 129.3

Fat: 7.7

Carbs: 10.1

Proteins: 6.5

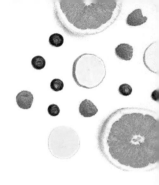
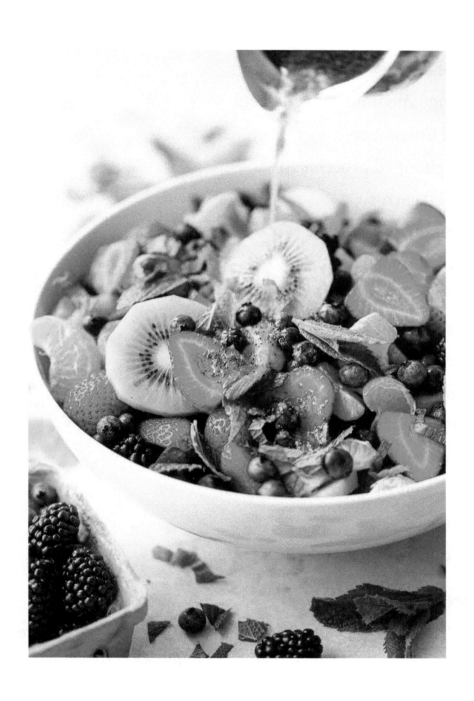

# Cucumber salad

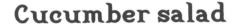
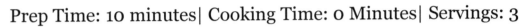

Prep Time: 10 minutes| Cooking Time: 0 Minutes| Servings: 3

## INGREDIENTS:

- 8 Cups of Mache
- 2 Julienned medium cooked beets,
- ½ Sliced Cucumber
- 1 Cup of chopped broccoli
- 1 Shredded carrot
- ½ Julienned, Bell pepper
- ¼ Cup of chopped almonds
- Ingredients to make the Almond Vinaigrette
- 4 Tablespoons of almond butter
- ¼ Tablespoon of olive oil
- 2 Tablespoons of freshly squeezed lemon juice
- 1 Tablespoon of raw honey
- ½ Minced garlic clove
- 2 Tablespoons of white wine vinegar
- 1 Pinch of sea salt
- 1 Pinch of freshly ground black pepper

## DIRECTIONS:

1. Into a deep bowl, combine your ingredients to make the almond vinaigrette; then whisk very well until your ingredients are very well mixed
2. Assemble your salad by mixing the ingredients altogether very well, except for the almonds
3. Drizzle your vinaigrette over your salad and toss the ingredients very well.

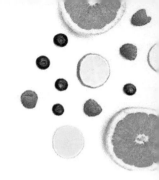

4. Top your salad with the chopped almonds

5. Serve and enjoy your salad!

**NUTRITION**

Kcal: 185

Fat: 14.7

Carbs: 10.6

Proteins: 0.81

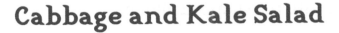

# Cabbage and Kale Salad

Prep Time: 10 minutes| Cooking Time: 0 Minutes| Servings: 2-3

## INGREDIENTS:

- 1 Cup of shredded green cabbage
- ½ Cup of shredded red cabbage
- 2 Cups of shredded raw kale
- 2 Shredded carrots
- 1 Cored, peeled and thinly sliced apple
- ¼ Cup of slivered almonds
- ¼ Cup of fresh blueberries
- ¼ Cup of extra virgin olive oil
- 2 Tablespoons of apple cider vinegar
- 2 Tablespoons of raw honey
- 1 Tablespoon of lemon juice
- 1 Pinch of sea salt
- 1 Pinch of freshly ground black pepper

## DIRECTIONS:

1. In a deep salad bowl, combine the green cabbage with the red cabbage, the carrots, the kale, the apple, and the blueberries.
2. Into a small bowl, mix the olive oil, the apple cider vinegar, the honey
3. Add the lemon juice; the salt and the pepper
4. Drizzle your vinaigrette over the salad and toss very well until your ingredients are very well blended
5. Top your salad with slivered almonds
6. Serve and enjoy your salad!

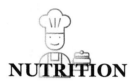

# NUTRITION

Kcal: 71

Fat: 3.6

Carbs: 9

Proteins: 2.1

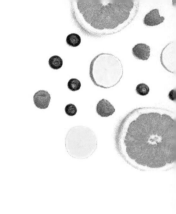

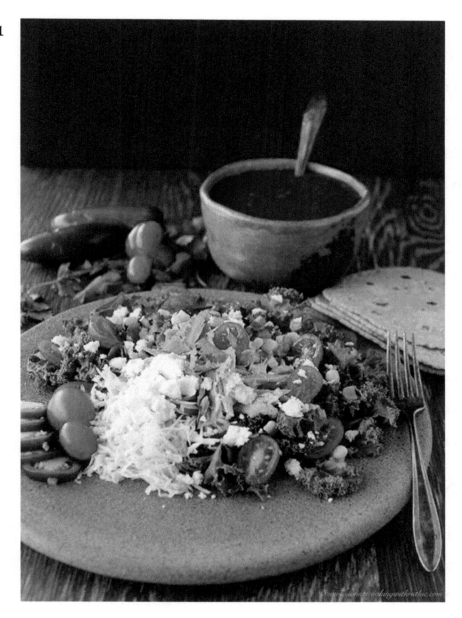

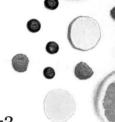

# Cranberry Salad

Prep Time: 10 minutes| Cooking Time: 0 Minutes| Servings: 2-3

## INGREDIENTS

To make the dressing:

- ¾ Cup of coconut milk Greek Yogurt
- ¼ Cup of honey
- 2 Tablespoons of apple cider vinegar
- 1 Pinch of salt
- 1 Pinch of freshly ground black pepper

To make the Coleslaw:

- 1 Small shredded cabbage
- 1 and ½ cups of matchstick carrots
- 2 Large sliced gala apples
- ½ Cup of sliced green onions
- ¾ Cup of slivered almonds
- ¾ Cup of dried cranberries

## DIRECTIONS:

1. Into a large mixing bowl; mix altogether the yogurt with the honey, the apple cider vinegar
2. Season with 1 pinch of salt and 1 pinch of pepper
3. In a deep and large bowl; toss altogether the cabbage, the carrots, the apples, the green onions, the almonds and the cranberries
4. Pour the dressing over the mixture of the cabbage

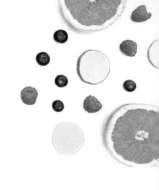

5. Toss your ingredients very well

6. Serve and enjoy your salad!

## NUTRITION

Kcal: 175

Fat: 11.1

Carbs: 16.6

Proteins: 5.2

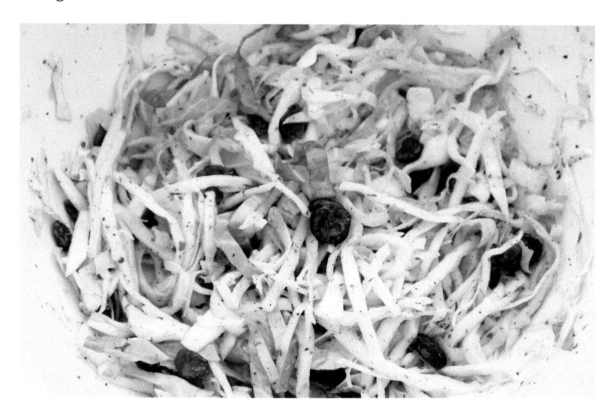

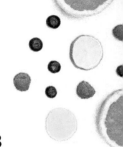

# Avocado and lettuce salad

Prep Time: 8 minutes| Cooking Time: 0 Minutes| Servings: 3

## INGREDIENTS

- ½ Torn green oak lettuce
- ½ Diced avocado
- 1 Large chopped mango
- 2 Tablespoons of toasted slivered almonds
- 2 Tablespoons of dried cranberries
- 1 Tablespoon of olive oil
- 1 Tablespoon of white wine vinegar

## DIRECTIONS:

1. Combine the lettuce with the avocado, the mango, the almonds and the cranberries into a deep and large bowl.
2. Whisk the oil and the vinegar altogether in a small bowl
3. Add a pinch of salt and a pinch of pepper.
4. Pour the seasoning over the mixture of the lettuce.
5. Toss the ingredients of the salt very well to combine it
6. Serve and enjoy your salad!

## NUTRITION

Kcal: 373.6

Fat: 19.8

Carbs: 8.7

Proteins: 5.6

# Pear and pumpkin seeds

Prep Time: 10 minutes| Cooking Time: 0 Minutes| Servings: 3

## INGREDIENTS:

- 1 Sliced and cored apple
- 1 Sliced and cored pear
- ½ Pound of sliced, hulled strawberries
- 2 Tablespoons of pumpkin seeds
- 8 Oz of spinach Leaves
- Ingredients to make the Strawberry Poppy seed Vinaigrette:
- ¼ Cup of cold filtered water
- ¼ Cup of olive oil
- ¼ Cup of red wine vinegar
- ½ Pound of hulled and sliced fresh strawberries
- 2 Tablespoons of honey
- ½ Teaspoon of poppy seeds

## DIRECTIONS:

1. Into a food processor, combine about ¼ cup of olive oil with ¼ cup of water, ¼ cup of cider vinegar

2. Add ½ Pound of strawberries and 2 tablespoons of honey; then puree the ingredients until it becomes smooth

3. Add about ½ teaspoon of poppy seeds and process very well to combine

4. Refrigerate the dressing into the refrigerator for about 15 minutes

5. Place your ingredients altogether into a large bowl; then add the dressing of the salad and combine very well

6. Serve and enjoy your salad!

**NUTRITION**

Kcal: 163

Fat: 9.6

Carbs: 14.9

Proteins: 5

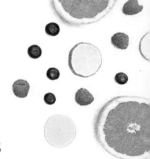

# Pomegranate Salad

Prep Time: 8 minutes| Cooking Time: 0 Minutes| Servings: 3

## INGREDIENTS

- 1 Medium, peeled and trimmed butternut squash
- 1 Pinch of salt
- 1 Pinch of pepper
- 1 large pear
- 5 oz of arugula
- ¾ Cup of pomegranate seeds
- ¾ Cup of roughly chopped walnuts
- To make the vinaigrette:
- 1 Tablespoon of maple syrup
- 1 Tablespoon of extra virgin olive oil
- 1 Tablespoon of sesame oil
- 2 Tablespoons of apple cider vinegar
- 1 Teaspoon of white sesame seeds
- 1 Tablespoon of coconut aminos
- 1 Pinch of pepper
- 1 Crushed and finely minced garlic clove

## DIRECTIONS:

1. Preheat your oven to a temperature of about 400° F
2. Line a baking sheet with a parchment paper; then lay the butternut squash
3. Lightly coat the squash with coconut oil; then season it with 1 pinch of salt and 1 pinch of pepper

4. Roast your ingredients for about 8 to 10 minutes

5. While your squash cooks is being cooked; mix your vinaigrette ingredients very well; then set it aside

6. Cut the pear into spirals; then add it to a mixing bowl

7. Add the walnuts and the arugula and once the butternut squash is perfectly cooked; transfer it to the your large bowl

8. Drizzle the vinaigrette and toss it very well

9. Serve and enjoy your salad!

**NUTRITION**

Kcal: 83.4

Fat: 3.8

Carbs: 12.02

Proteins: 3.5

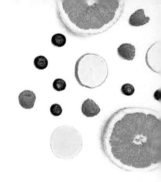

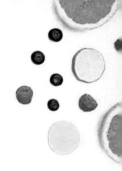